The Gift.

Root Chakra

Inspirational Quotes

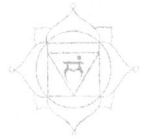

Written by Amirah Bellamy
Illustrations by Artabulous

The Gift: Root Chakra
Inspirational Quotes

is dedicated to the blessing of new beginnings.

Acknowledgments

I thank the divine essence within for being the grounding force that empowers me to continue.

Opening Remarks...

We wrote the second series of "The Gift" with the intention of inspiring you to enjoy the glorious gift of balanced and free flowing chakras. Chakras are the sacred energy centers within your body, which more simply stated is invisible life force energy that keeps you vibrant, healthy and alive. Thus, each page in this book includes inspirational quotes gathered from the depths of our own divine inspiration that focuses on the essence of each of the 7 main chakras. As always, we have written this book in the pure, positive spirit of love in the hopes that you will enjoy it during pleasurable moments and use it to heal during difficult times.

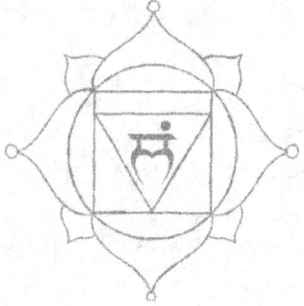

The beginning of your
story will always be
the best part.

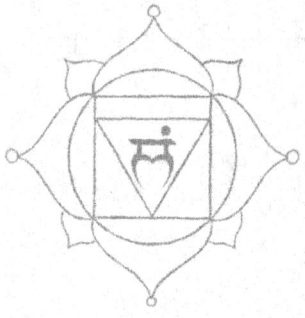

A strong
foundation makes
the weak spots
irrelevant .

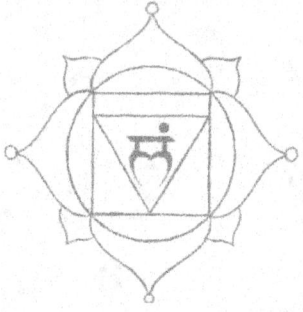

At your most basic

level you are

evolved.

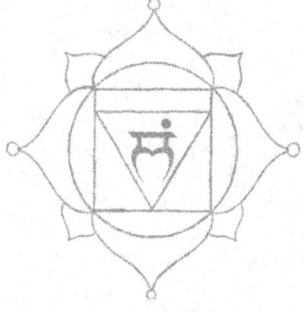

AT THE ROOT OF
EVERY PROBLEM
LIES THE
SOLUTION.

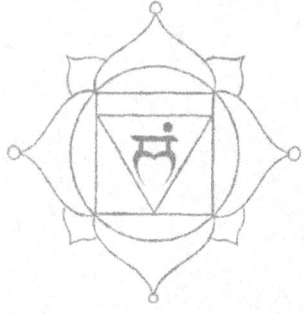

Being the pioneer

of **your** life makes

you the master of

all.

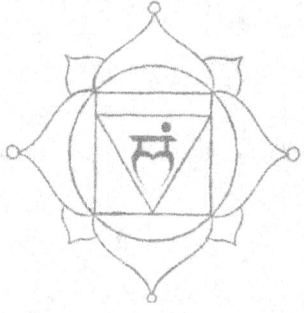

The evolution of
your story
depends on how
good the
beginning is and
you can always
start anew.

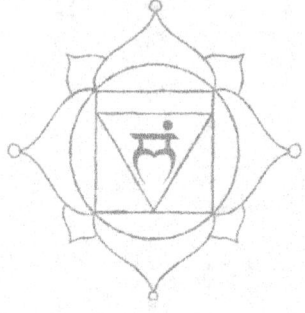

At your core you are
flawless.

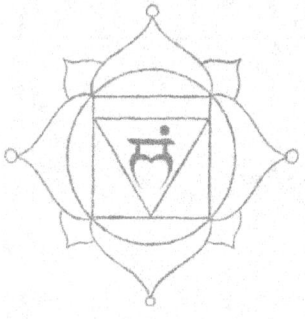

Though unseen the root
of who you are is your
very essence. It is your
genesis, your support,
your nourishment.

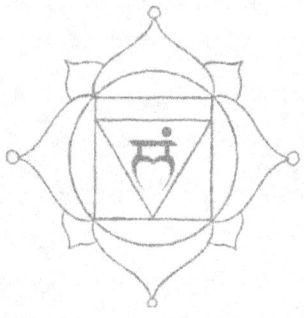

Let everyday begin as the best part of you and it will be the foundation that supports all of you.

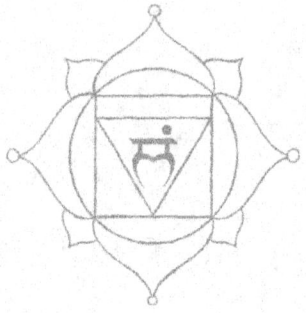

Stay grounded in
you and you will
remain firmly
rooted.

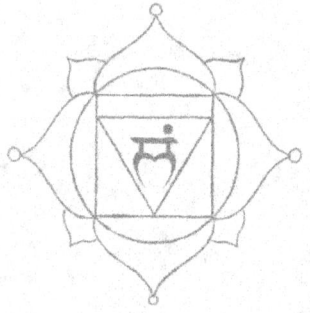

LOOK AT THE MOST

BASIC ASPECTS OF

YOURSELF TO FIND THE

MOST BEAUTIFUL

CONFIRMATIONS.

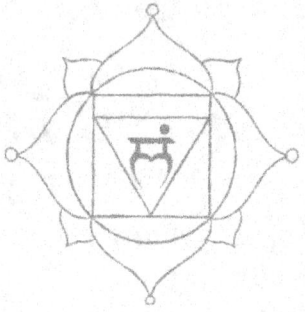

The truth is...

The essence of you is

divine, loving and joyful.

Be the real you...

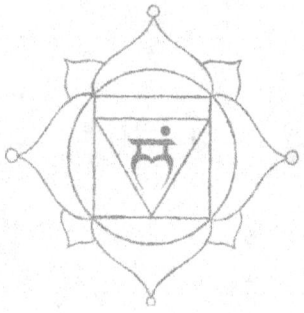

YOU are Here TO
realize THE
FreeDOM TO Grow
into someone
JOYOUSLY
BeaUTIFUL.

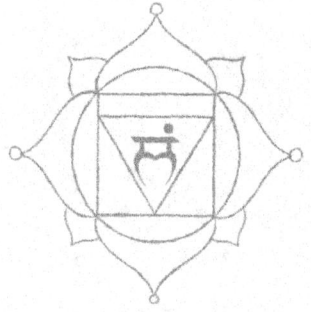

If life causes you
to rebuild it is
because you are a
masterful builder.

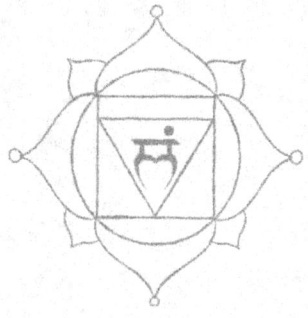

The existence of you if very purposefully grounded and rooted in life's source.

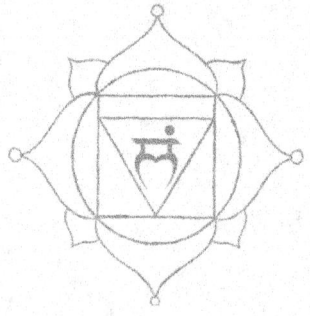

What the eye can
see of you is
minuscule.

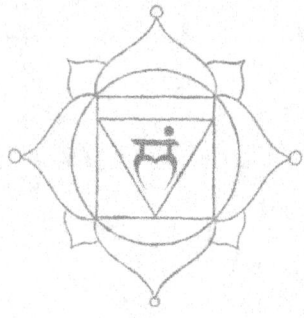

when you are
grounded in *your*
truth you are most
firmly rooted at the
height of your
expansion.

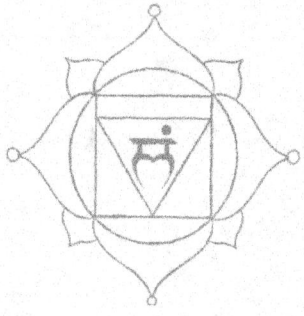

Naturally you are
an organized body
of knowledge, the
science that baffles
the mind.

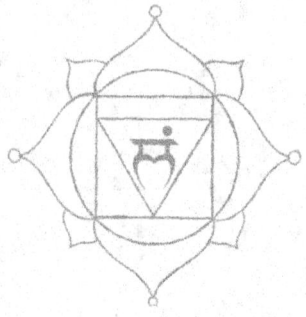

The more you expand,
the more you return to
the *source* of your
beginning.

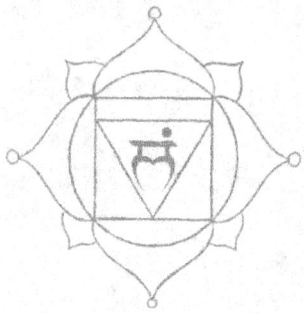

Life...

is an adventure that

begins and ends with

you.

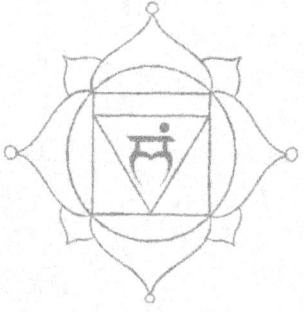

The intricacies of you barely touch the surface of your depth.

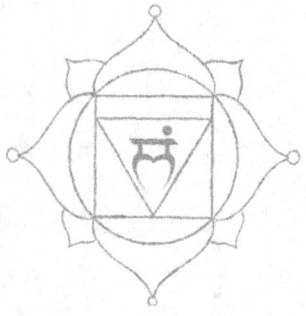

In your journey of
self-discovery
always go back to
the basics.

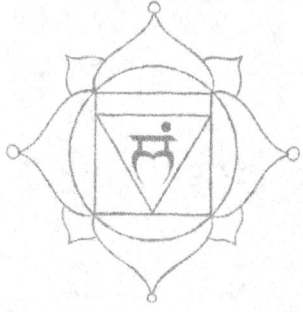

The breath is the entirety of
your being as you breathe new
life into each moment manifested
as a new opportunity.

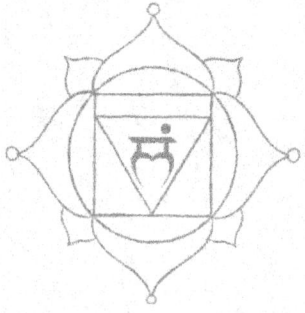

Like seasons you are forever changing into another phase of the continuous cycle of your expansion.

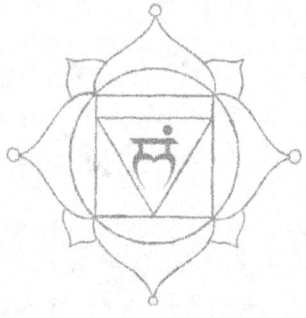

Fundamentally....
you are necessary.

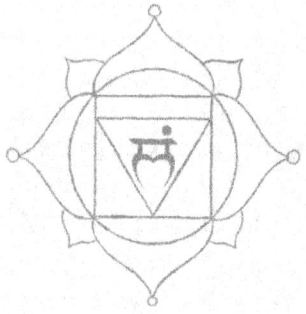

To truly know a

person you need

only have

awareness of their

roots.

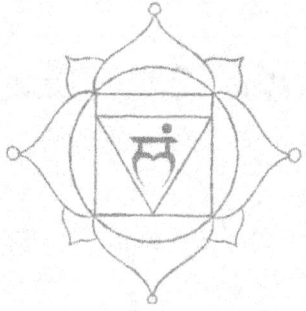

You are the matter that matters, the mass occupant of space continuously expanding into the fact that leaves no room for debate.

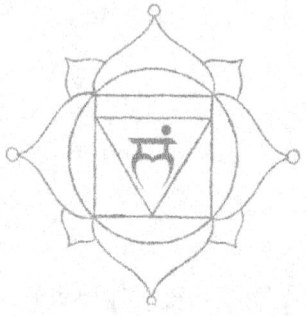

The best surprises in life
are the ones that are
always there.

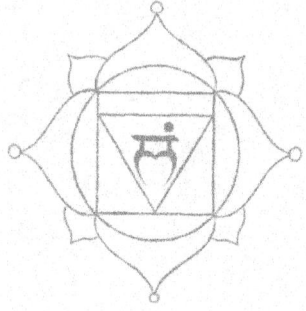

The peace that you seek lies
at the root of who you are.

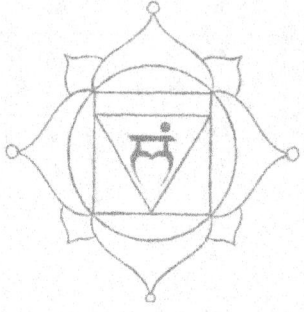

Begin each moment with
a new perspective of
delight.

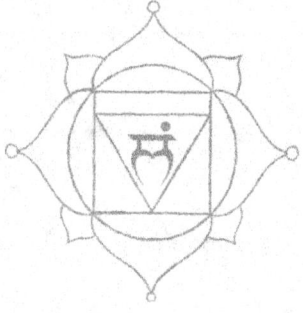

The most important
relationship is the one that
you have with yourself.
Stay committed to making
it glorious.

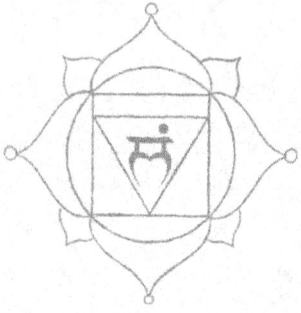

Out *of the darkness came*

the miracle of you.

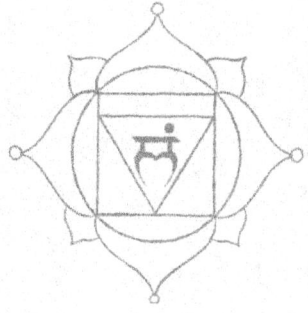

WHEN YOUR LIFE IS
CONSUMED WITH
DARKNESS IT IS TIME
TO CULTIVATE
SOMETHING
ENLIGHTENING
WITHIN.

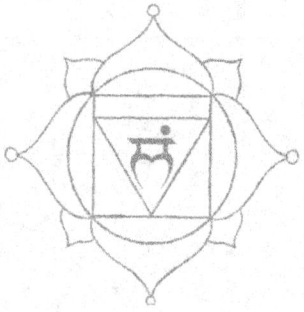

Within you lies the power of *creation.* Create.

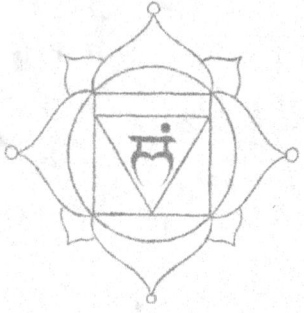

You always have the fortitude to be more.

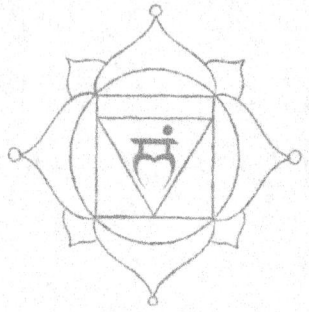

In the absence of your fear
lies the famed magician.

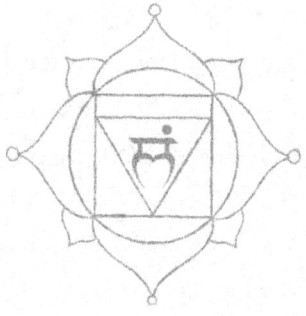

When there is only you,

honest is all that you can

be.

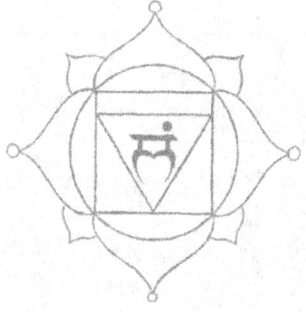

Free your doubts and
grow them into
dreams come true.

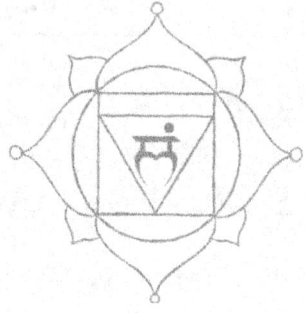

If you feel lost it is because
as you expand you become
a stranger to yourself.

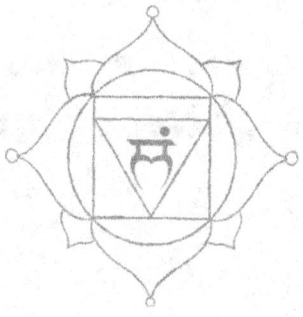

Expect the best in everyone and you will never be disappointed.

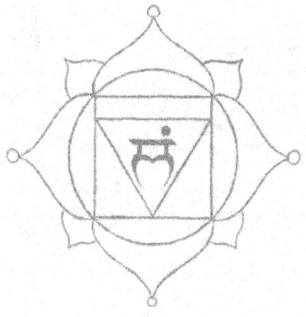

Sometimes the worst is the **BEST** *thing that could ever happen.*

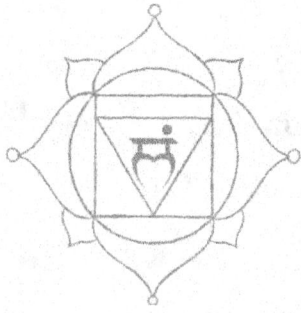

The Self is always the
highest order.

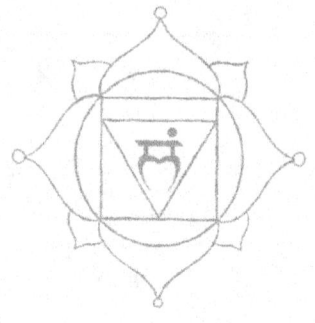

Be the cheering squad who is always

rooting for a wonderful cause....

YOU.

We hope that the quotes in this book were a healing, fulfilling medicine for your soul and that they in some way enriched your life. With that we wish you a life of love in abundance and a more blissful vision of the world.

Exist purely in love!

If you enjoyed this book or received value from it in any way, then I'd like to ask you for a favor. Would you be kind enough to leave a review for this book on Amazon? It'd be greatly appreciated!

About the Author...

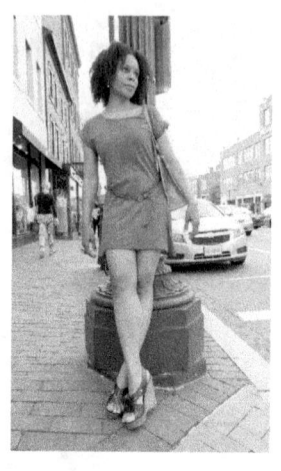

Amirah Bellamy is the Executive Board Chair of Life Arts Institute. She has a BS and MA in Counseling Psychology. She's also an artist of many crafts. She's been a writer for over 19 years, a yogi for over 10 years, a singer for over 15 years, nutritionista for over 16 years and has thoroughly enjoyed being mom to 2 beautiful children.

To learn more about Amirah Bellamy

visit..... www.EthericRealmsInv.com

Other books by this author....

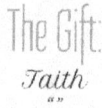

The Gift:
Faith
" "

Written by Amirah Bellamy
Illustrations by Artabulous

The Gift:
Happiness
" "

Written by Amirah Bellamy
Illustrations by Artabulous

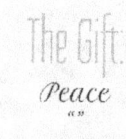

The Gift:
Peace
" "

Written by Amirah Bellamy
Photography by Jamari Bellamy

The Gift:
Gratitude
" "

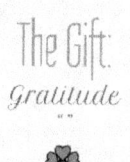

Written by Amirah Bellamy
Illustrations by Artabulous

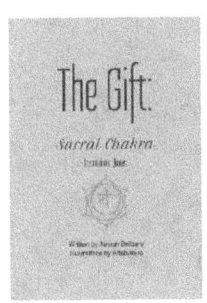

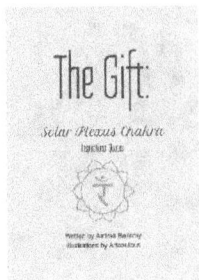

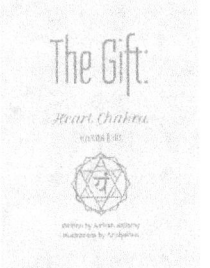

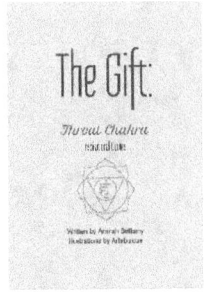

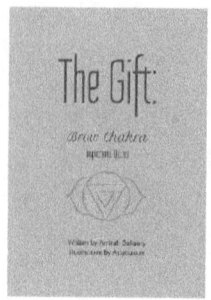

The Gift:

Brow Chakra

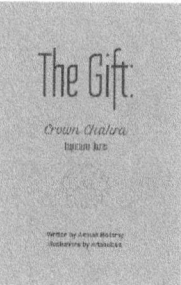

The Gift:

Crown Chakra